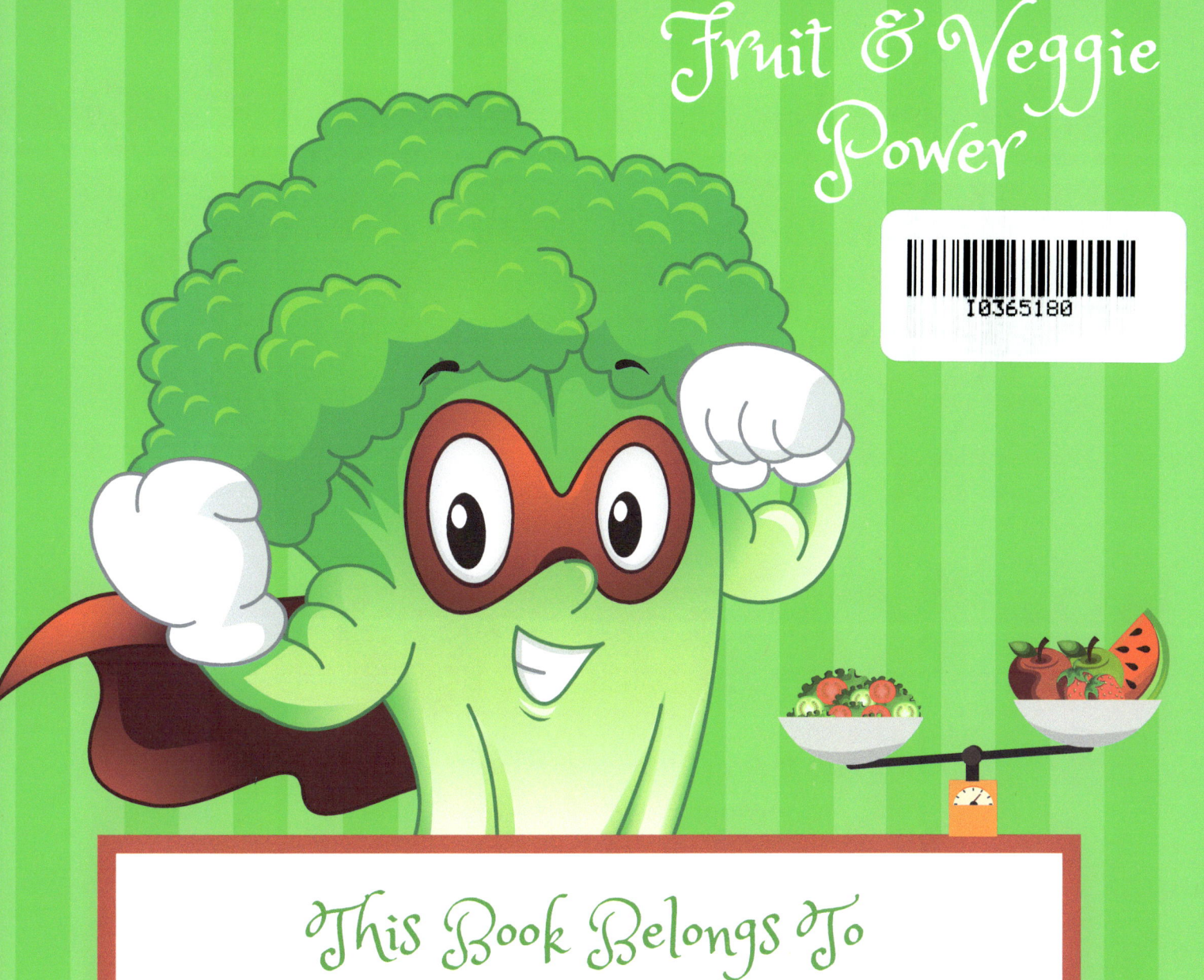

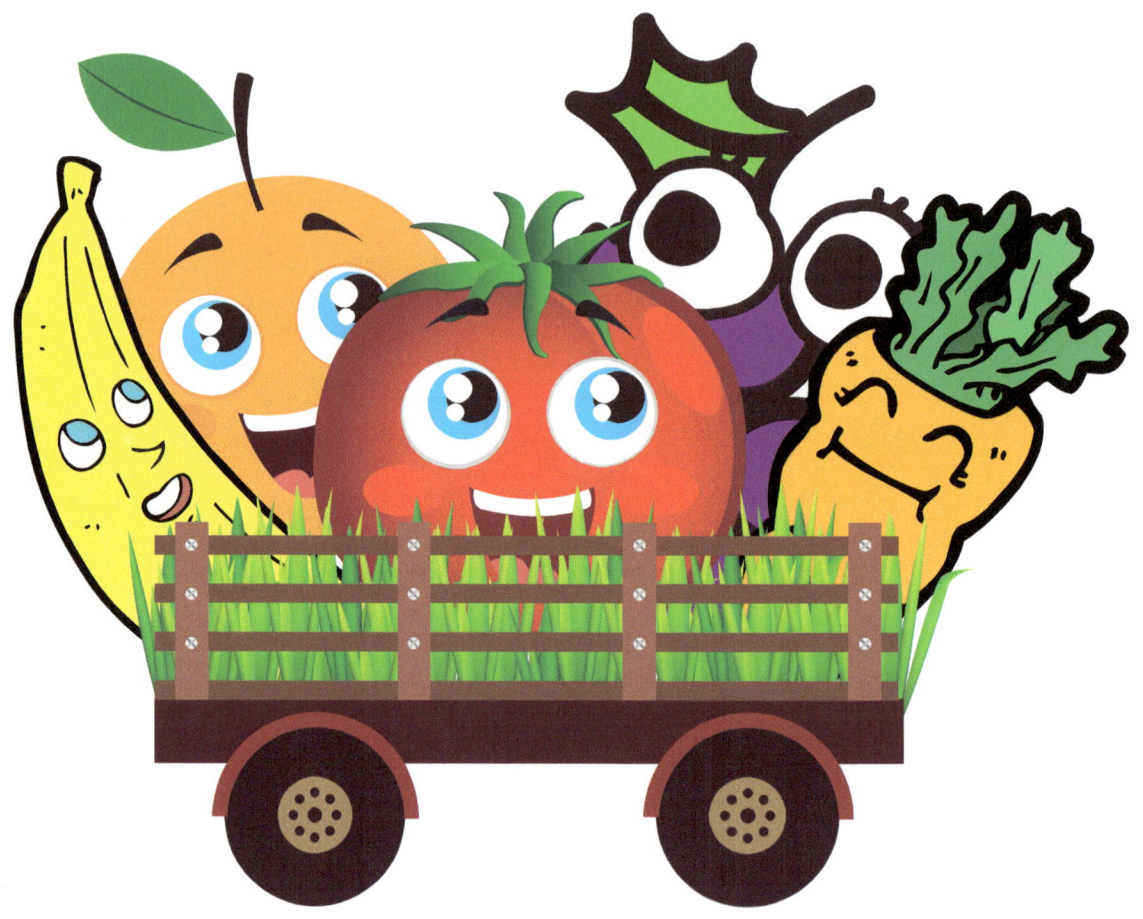

Let's Have A Fruity Good Time With Veggies

Copyright © 2019 by Tasana Scales

All Rights Reserved

Published by Tasana Scales. Some image credits to Shutterstock and Canva. Order copies at www.kidmotivation.com.

Printed in the United States of America

ISBN 978-1-7336490-3-2

Written & Designed by Tasana Scales

Dear Parents:

Encouraging kids to eat fruits and veggies promotes good health and protects against disease. There is strong evidence to show that the nutrients found in fruits and veggies strengthen a child's immune system and help fight illnesses. Fruits and veggies are rich in vitamins and minerals that help you feel healthy and energized. Visit us for more books at www.kidmotivation.com.

Pick One Today

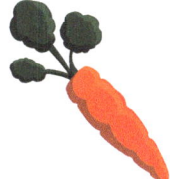 carrot   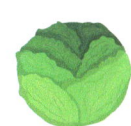 cabbage    banana

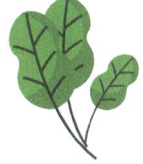 spinach   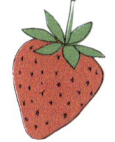 strawberry   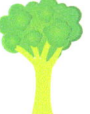 broccoli

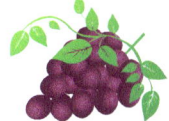 grapes   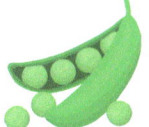 peas   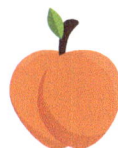 peach

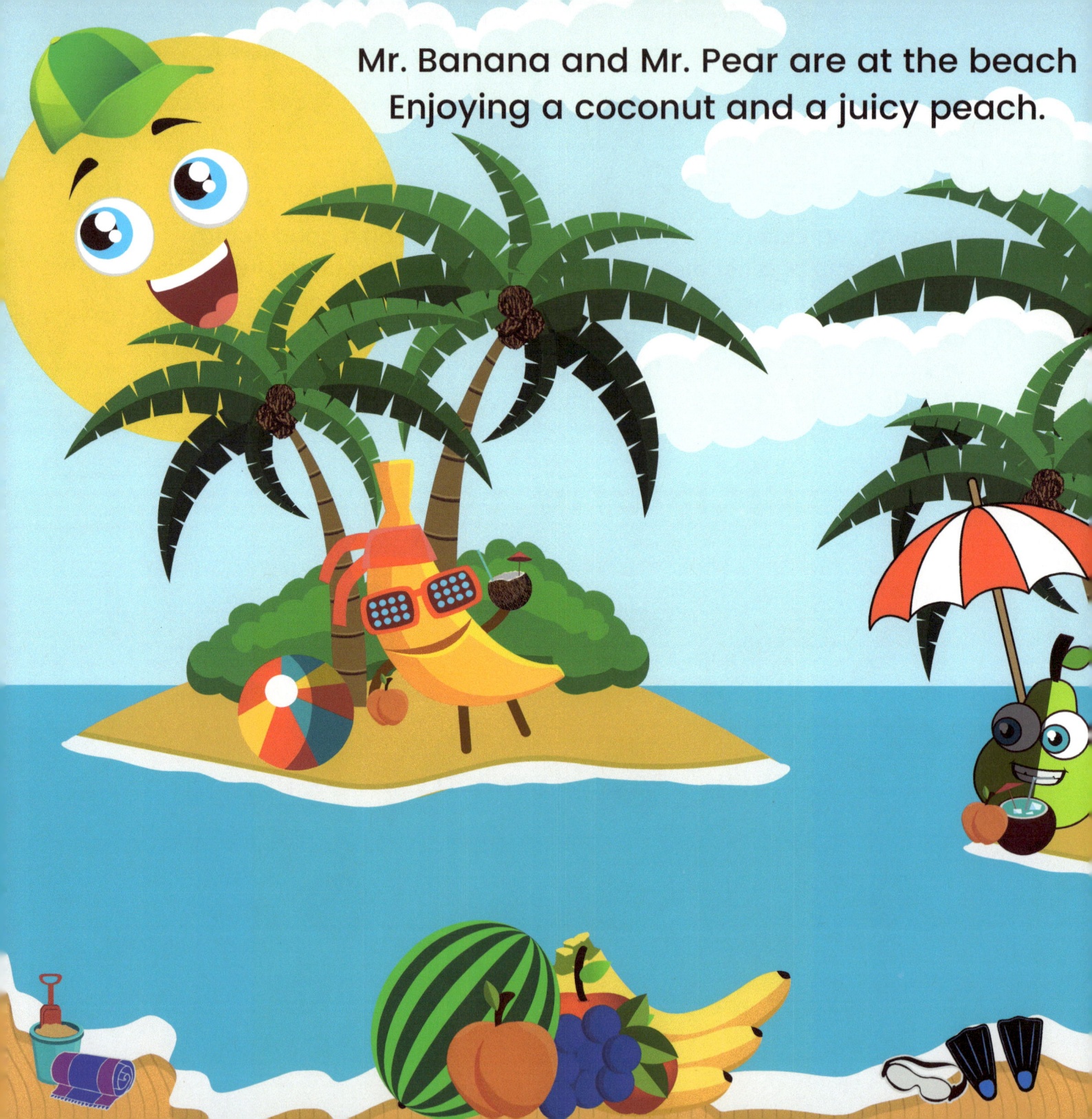

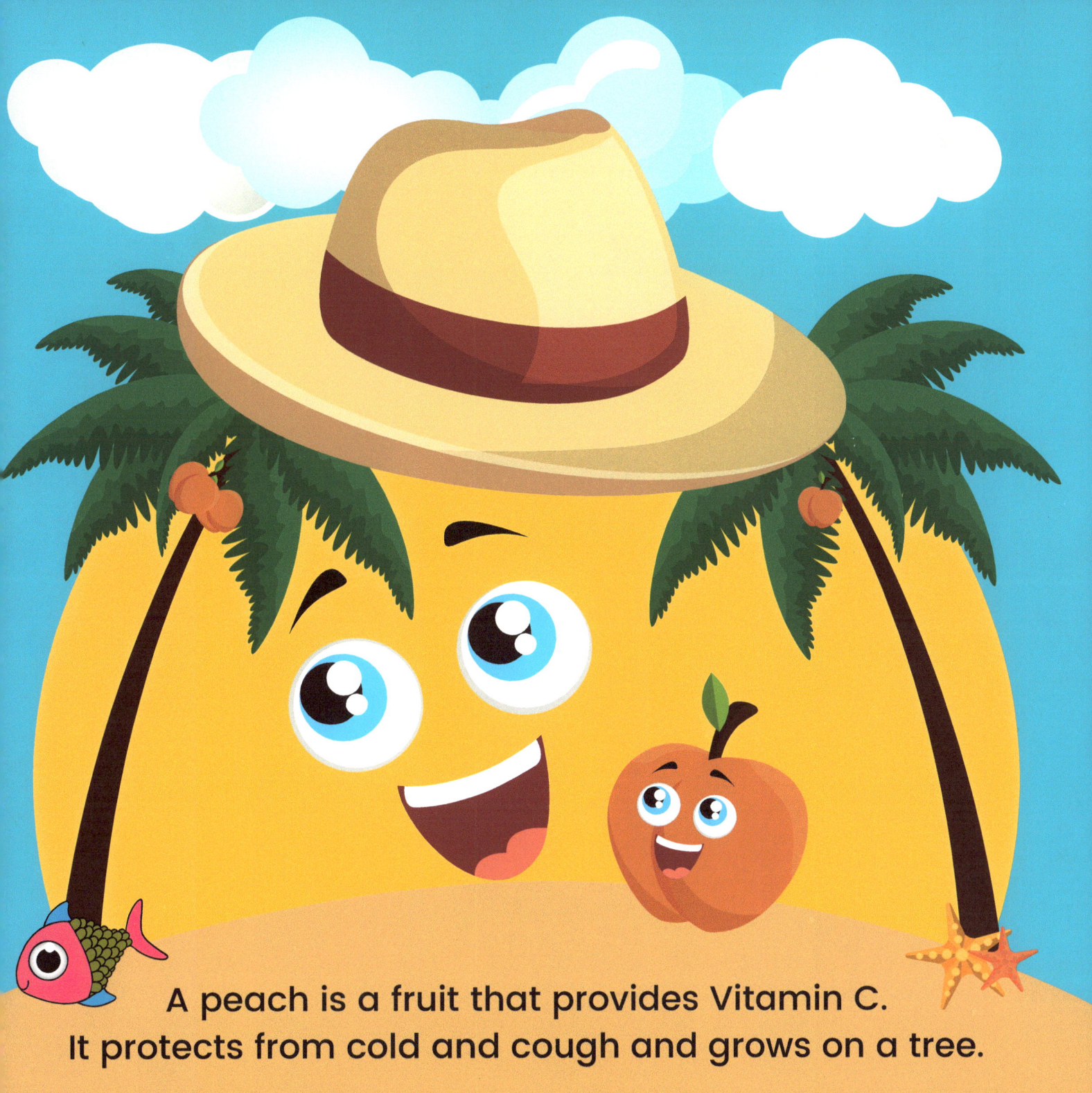

The Tomatoes went to the circus to laugh and play
And amazingly watch the elephant jump through the fire...
NO WAY!

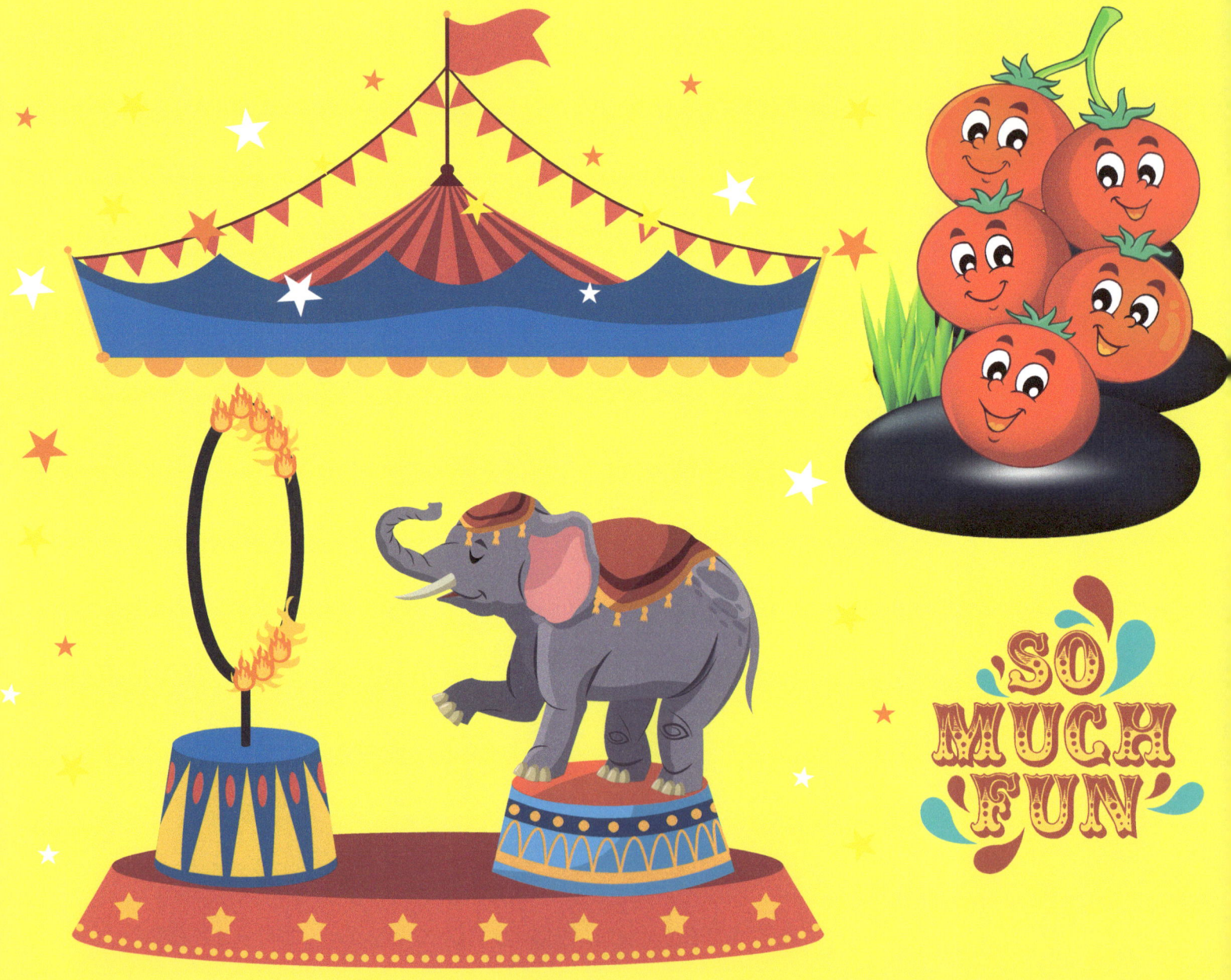

So Much Fun

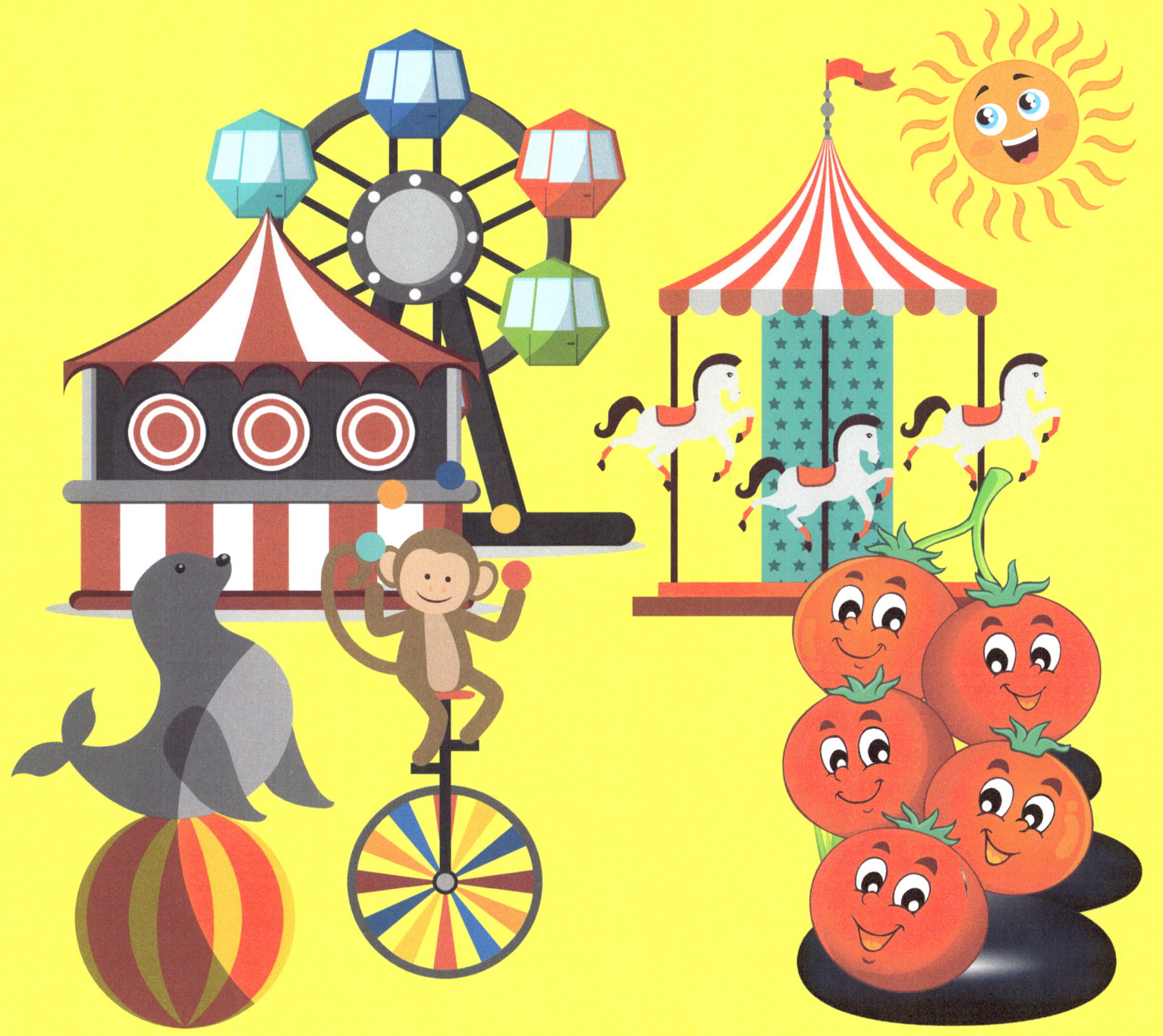

A Tomato is a fruit that grows on a vine.
It provides many vitamins and loves the sunshine.

Mr. Cucumber drove to church in his new car
Singing and dancing like a movie star.

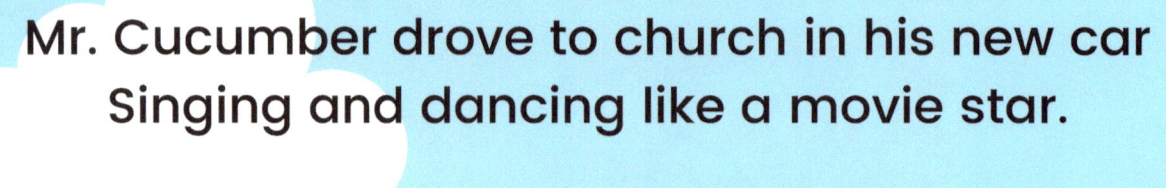

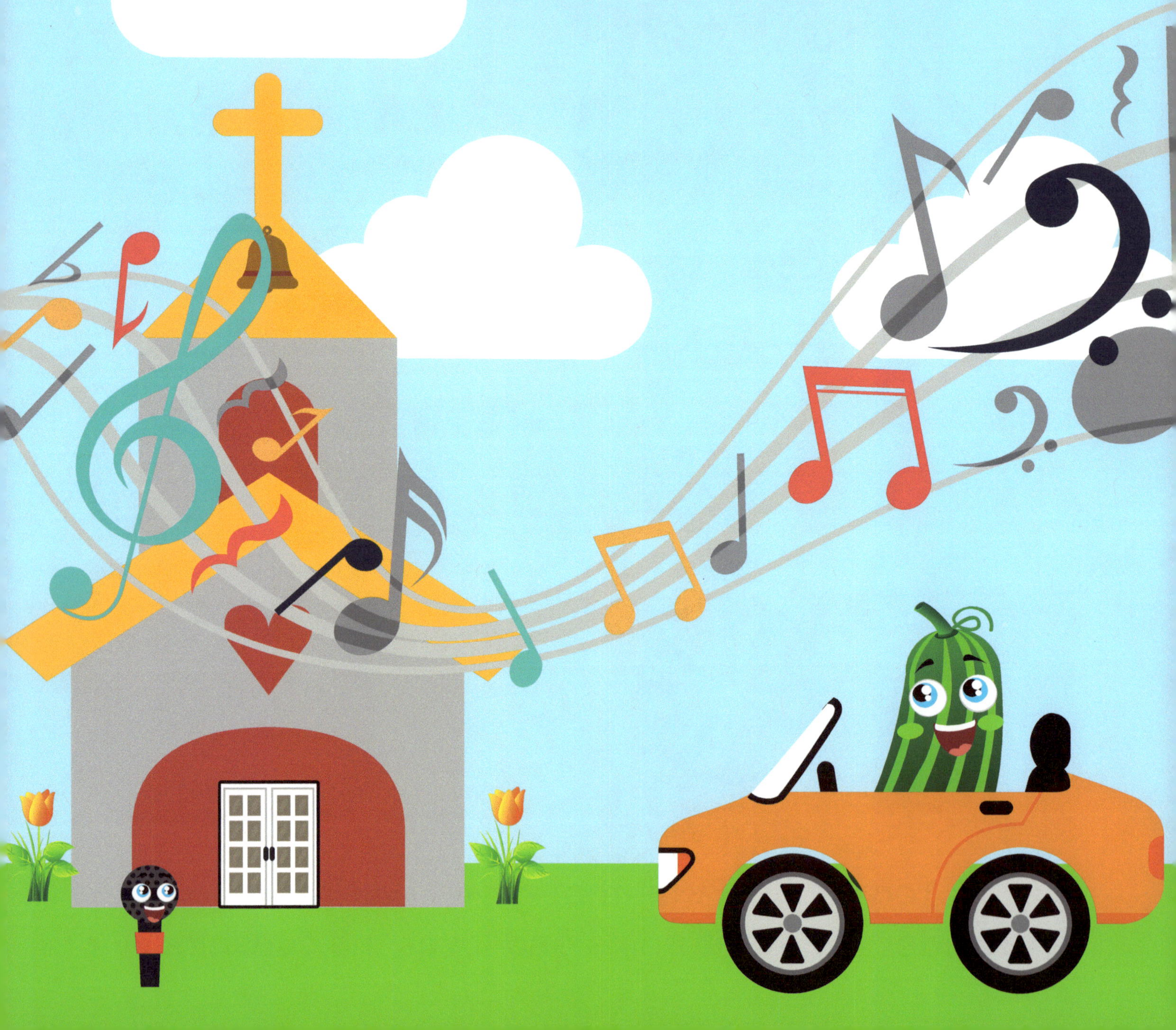

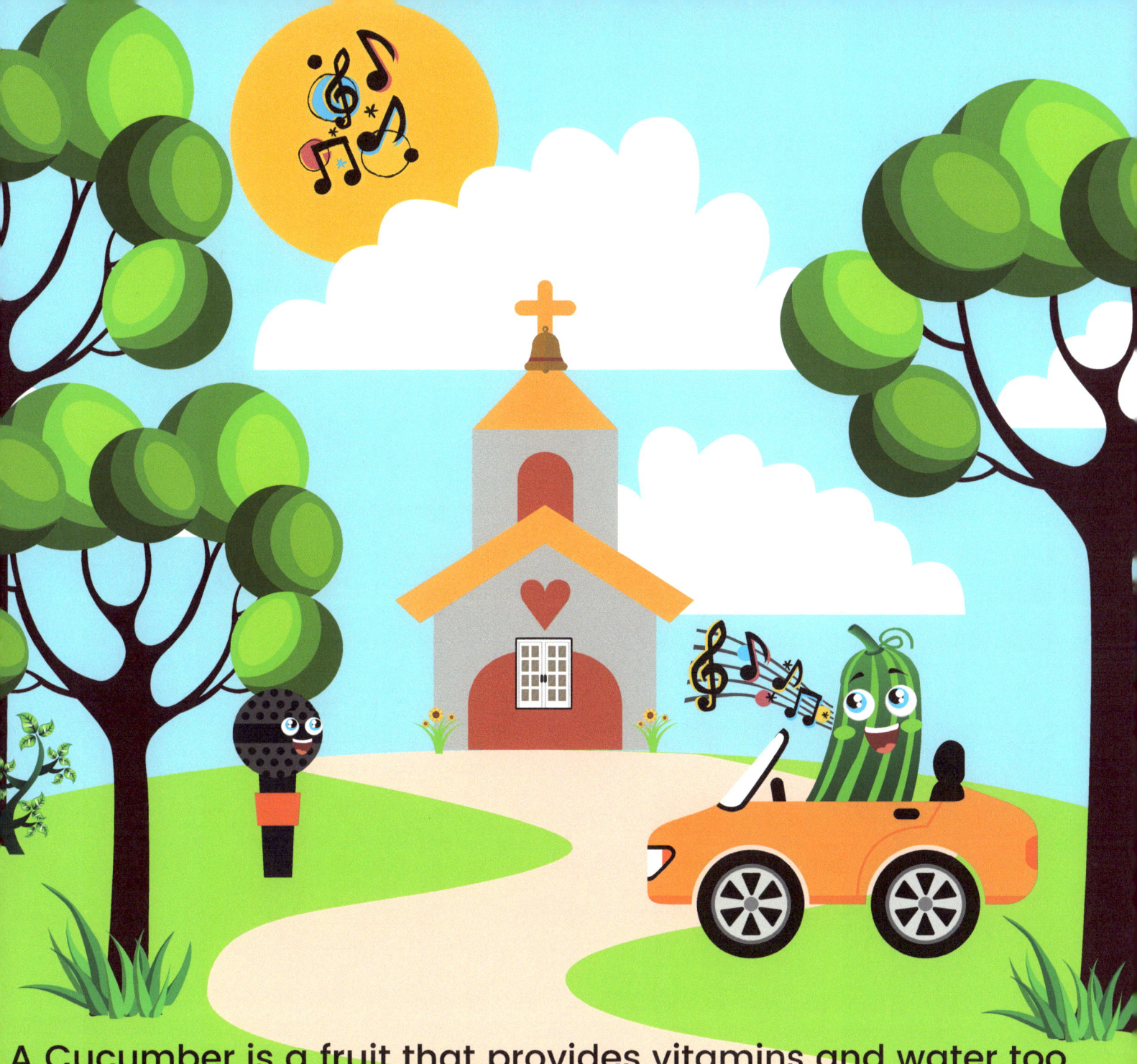

A Cucumber is a fruit that provides vitamins and water too.
It is green, it is healthy, it keeps the skin glowing and new.

Mr. Grapes and Mrs. Pear rode the train to town
Going up and around, going straight and then down.

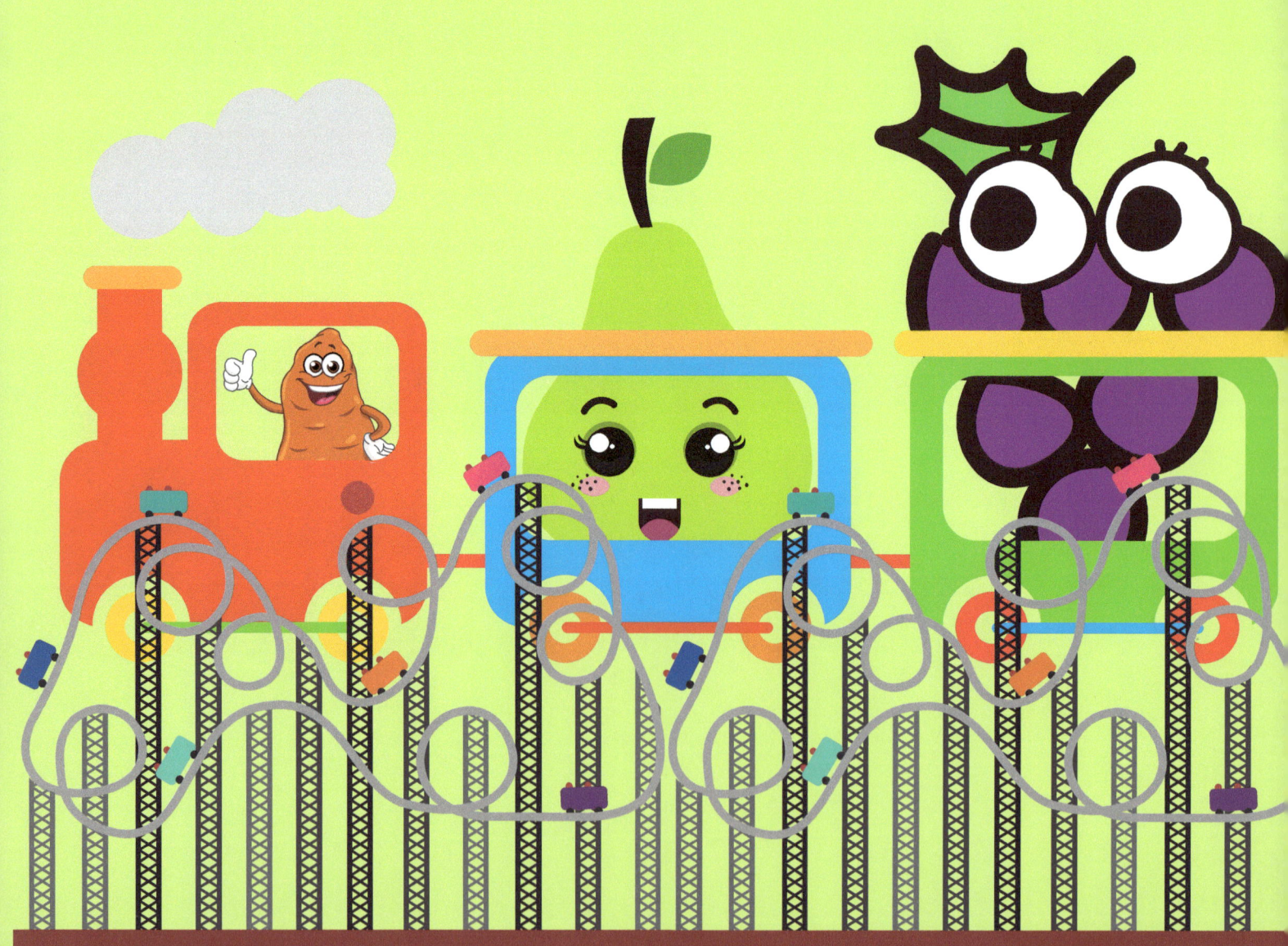

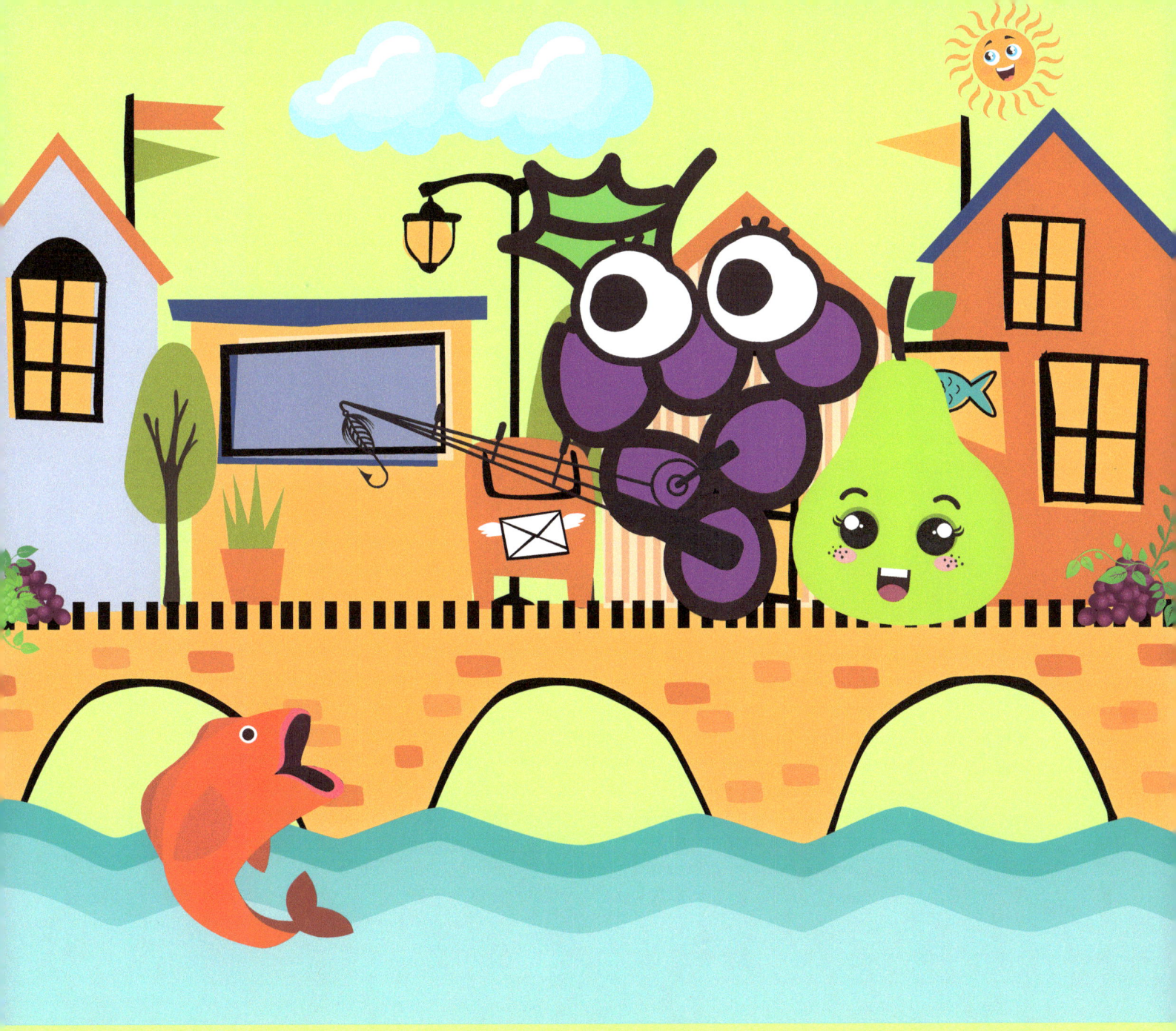

Grapes are fruit that provides Vitamin C.
It grows on a vine and is as sweet as can be.

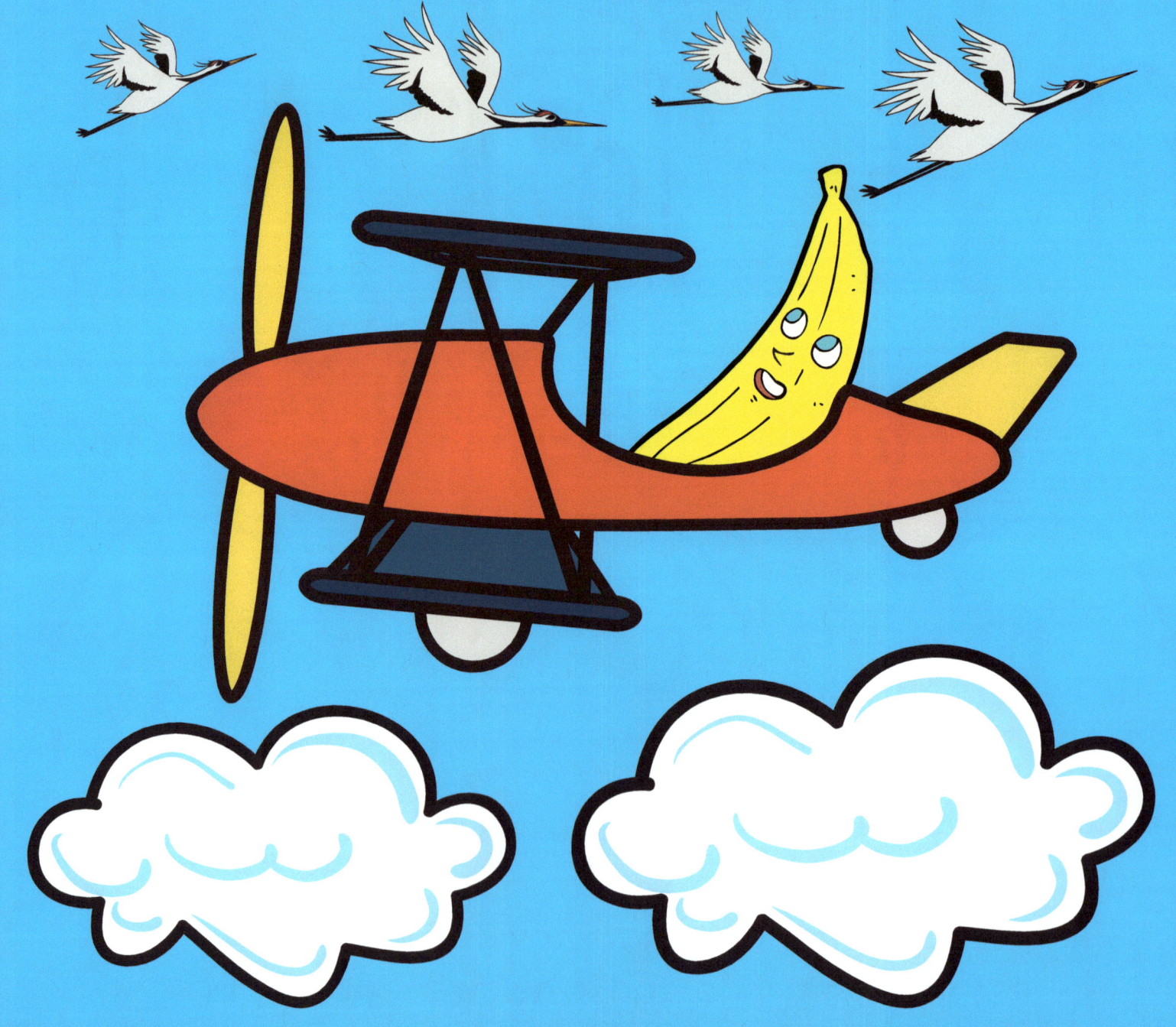

Mr. Banana is flying high in the blue sky
Above the clouds as birds are passing by.

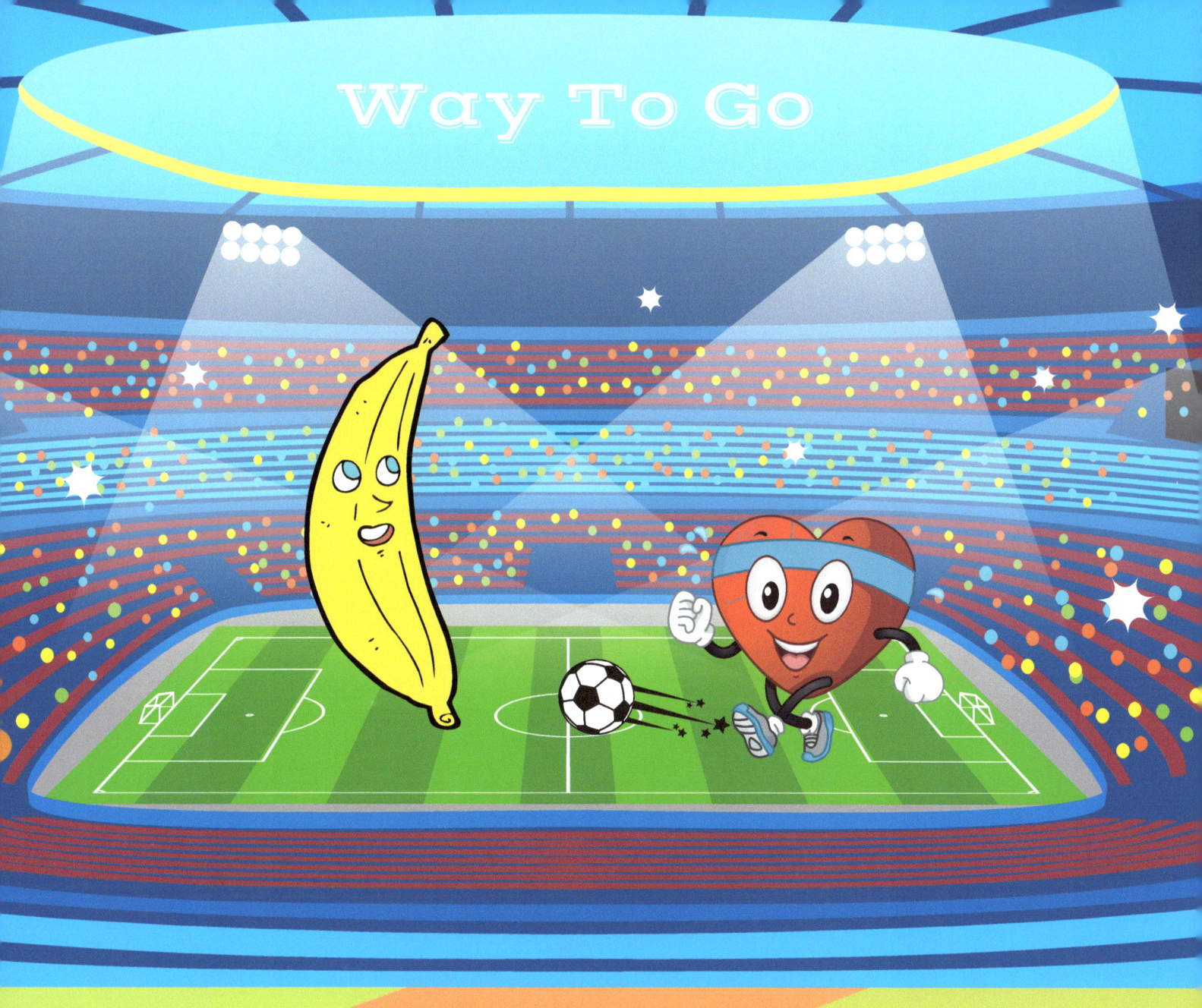

A banana is fruit that provides potassium and Vitamin C. It is yellow and great tasting and keeps the heart healthy.

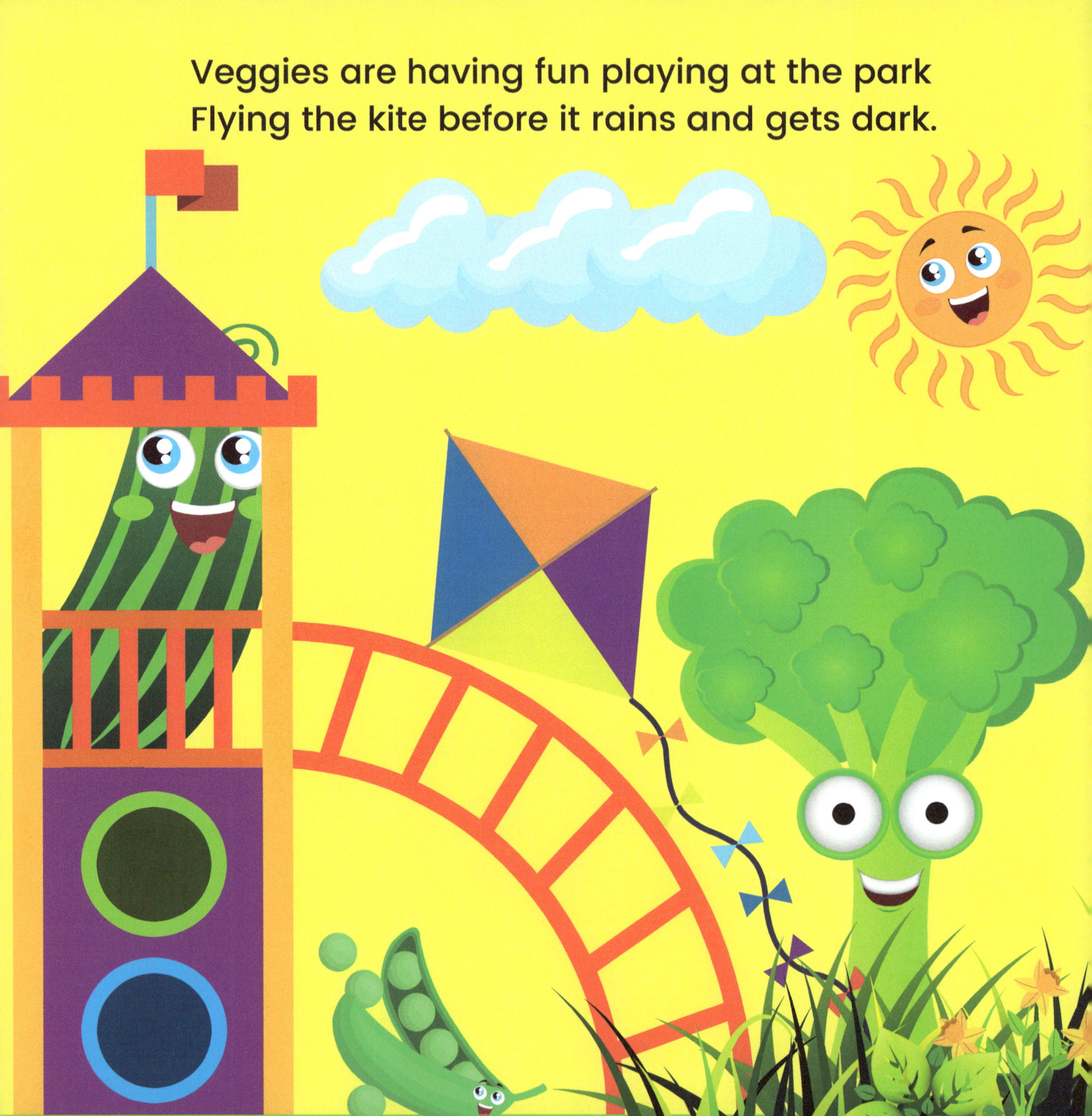

Veggies are having fun playing at the park
Flying the kite before it rains and gets dark.

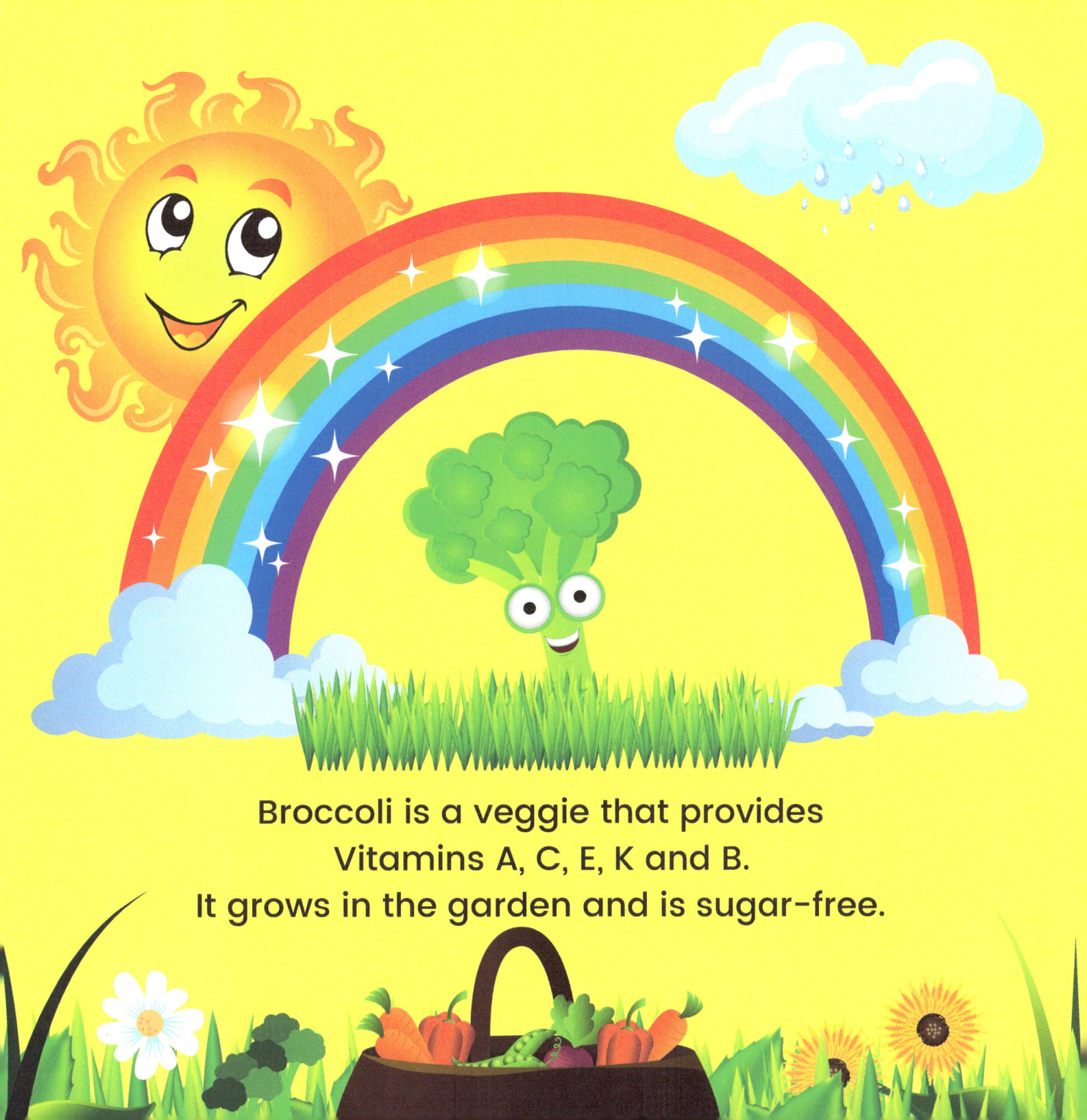

Broccoli is a veggie that provides
Vitamins A, C, E, K and B.
It grows in the garden and is sugar-free.

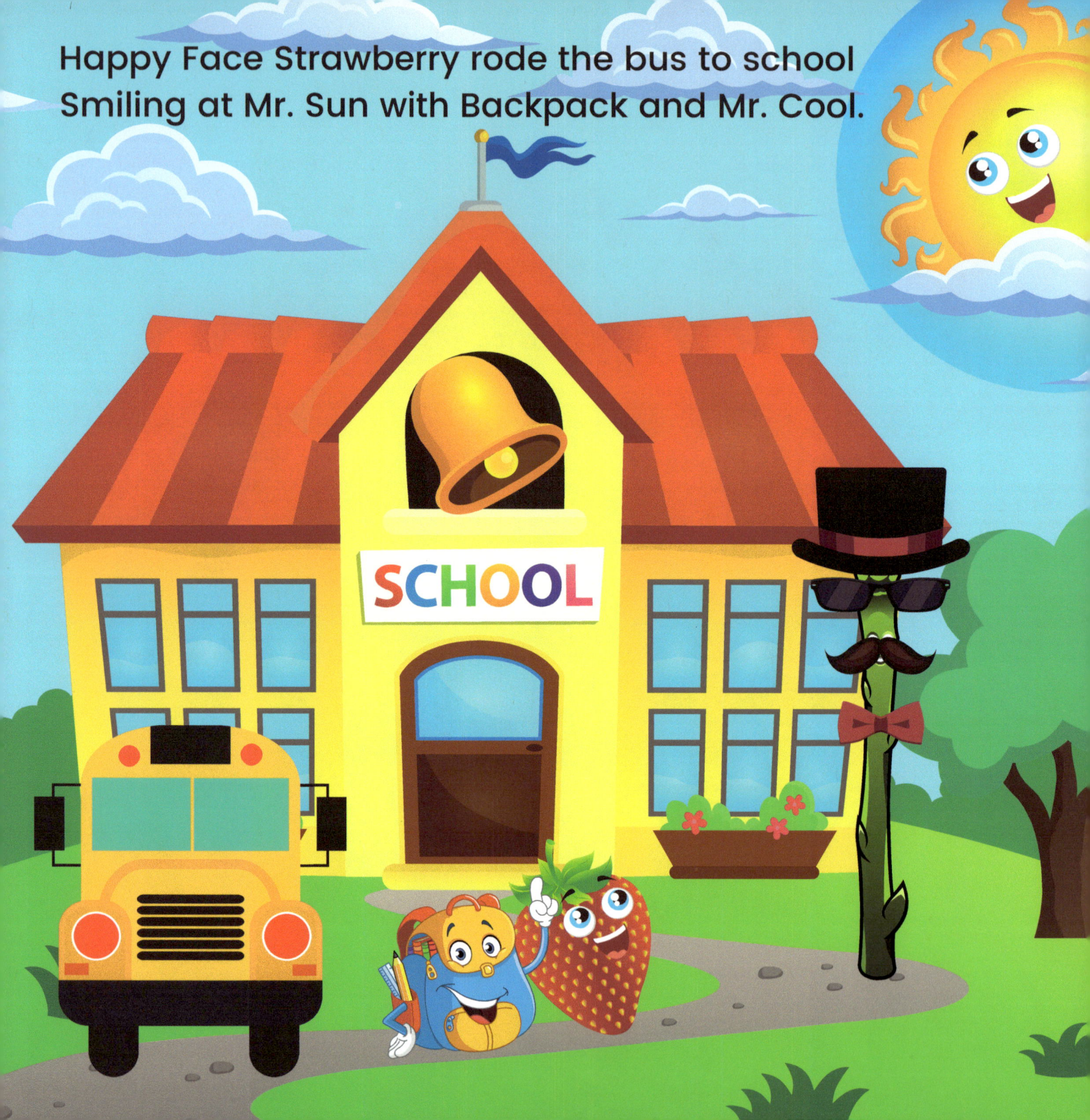
Happy Face Strawberry rode the bus to school Smiling at Mr. Sun with Backpack and Mr. Cool.

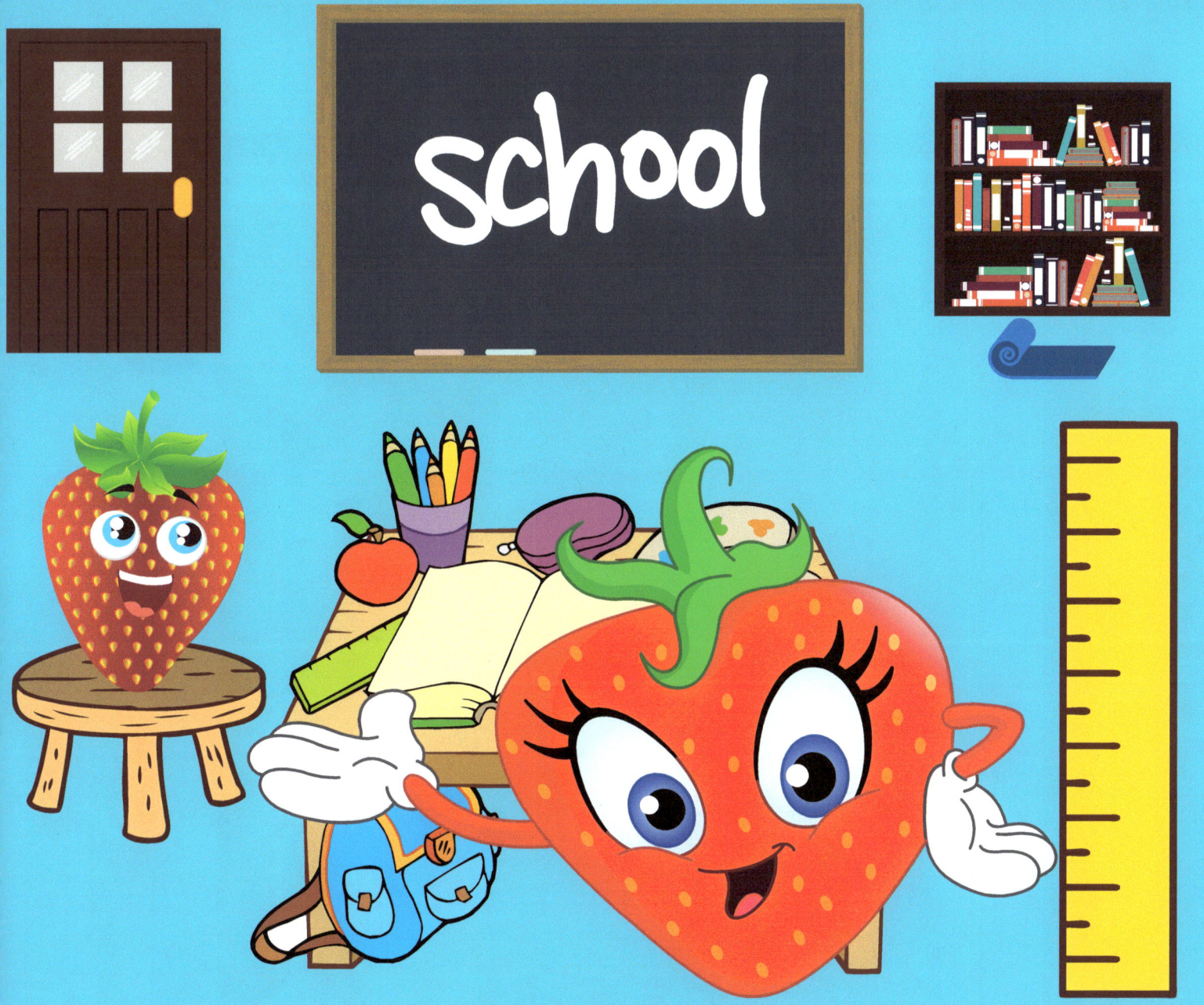

A strawberry is a fruit that provides Vitamin C.
It is red, it is juicy, and it is fat-free.

Mr. Orange followed the rocket to outer space
With his eyes wide open and a smile on his face.

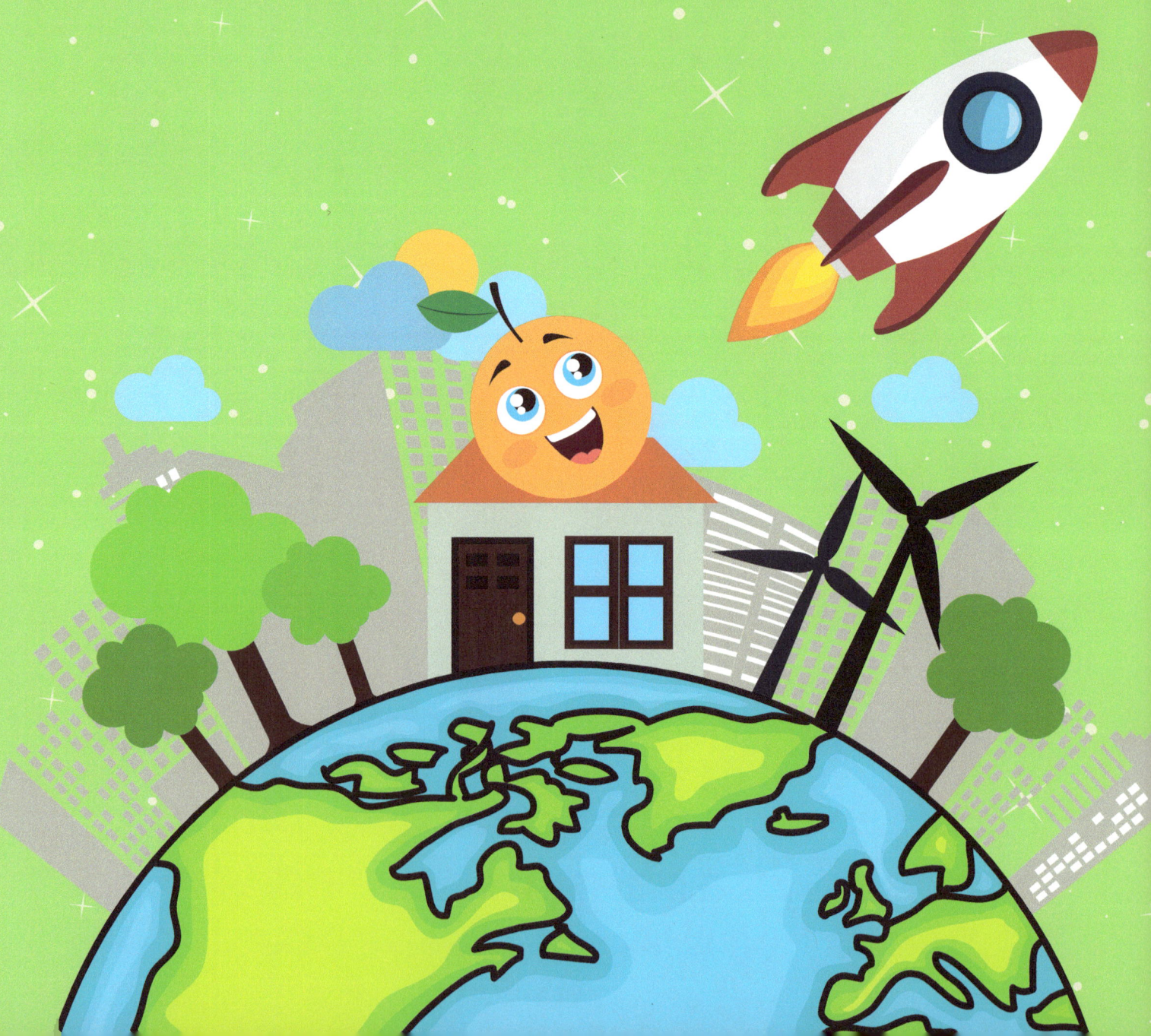

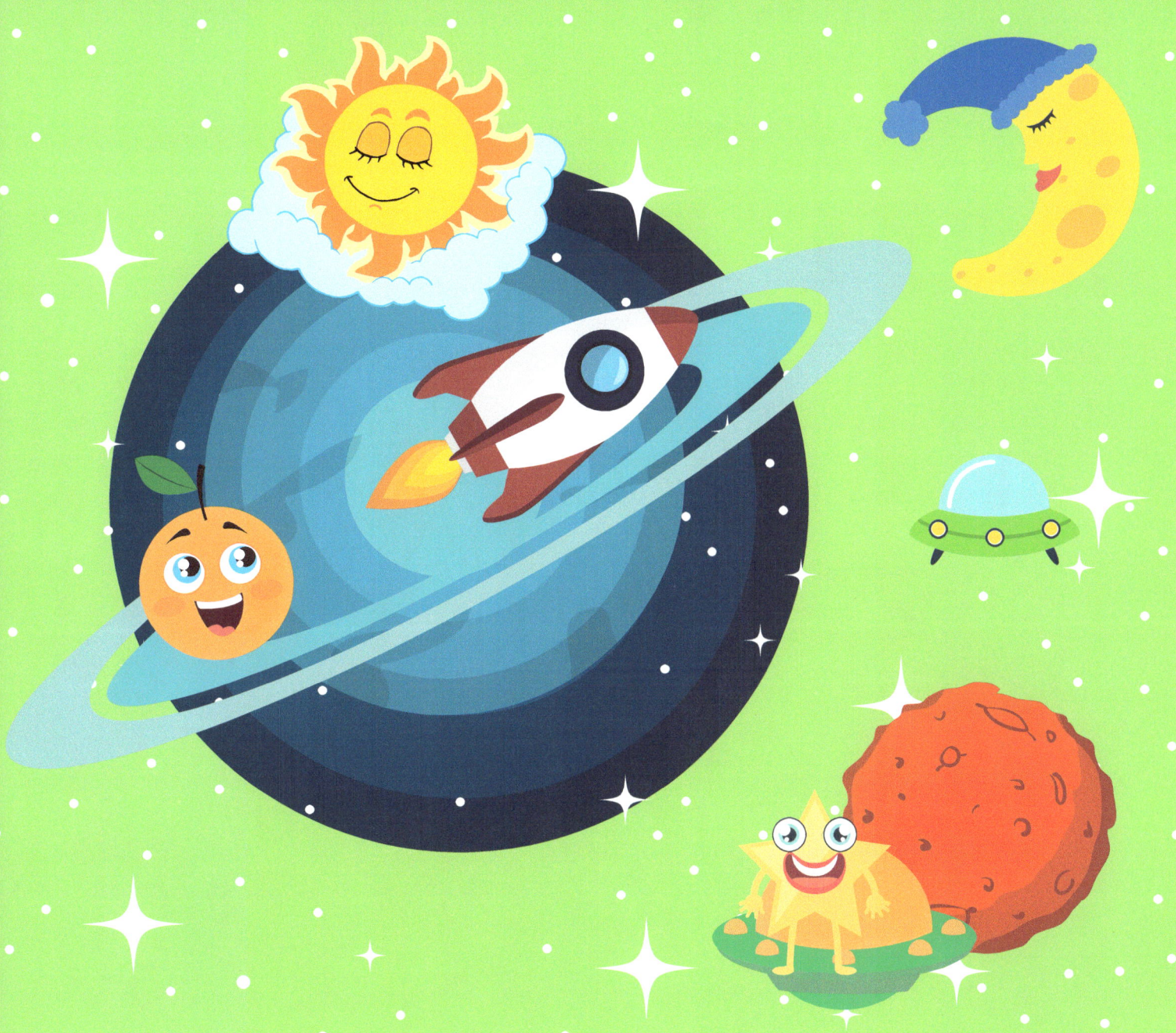

An orange is a fruit that provides Vitamin C.
It helps fight illnesses and keeps you healthy as can be.

Green Pear and Yellow Pear at home having fun
Enjoying the fresh air in the tree in the sun.

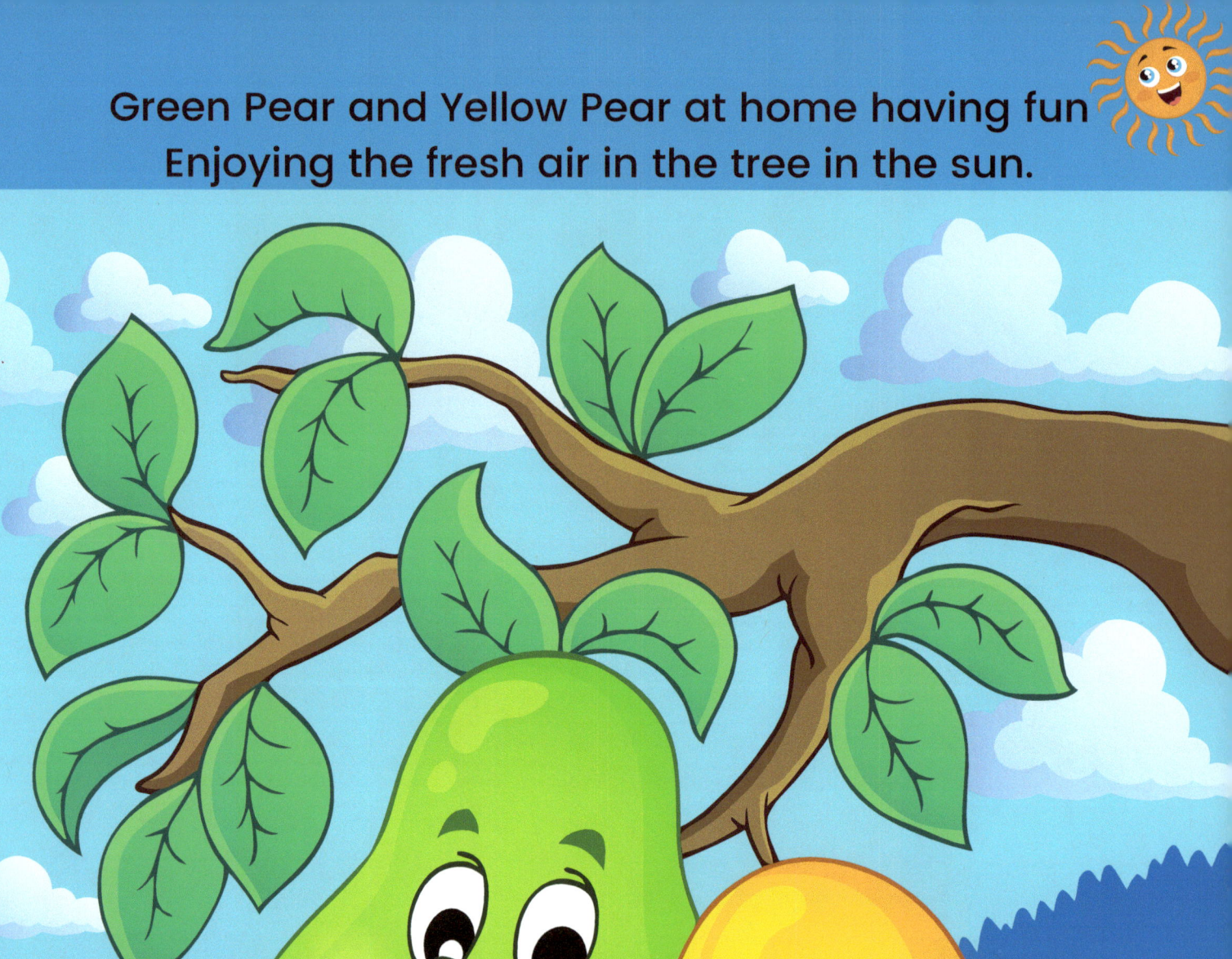

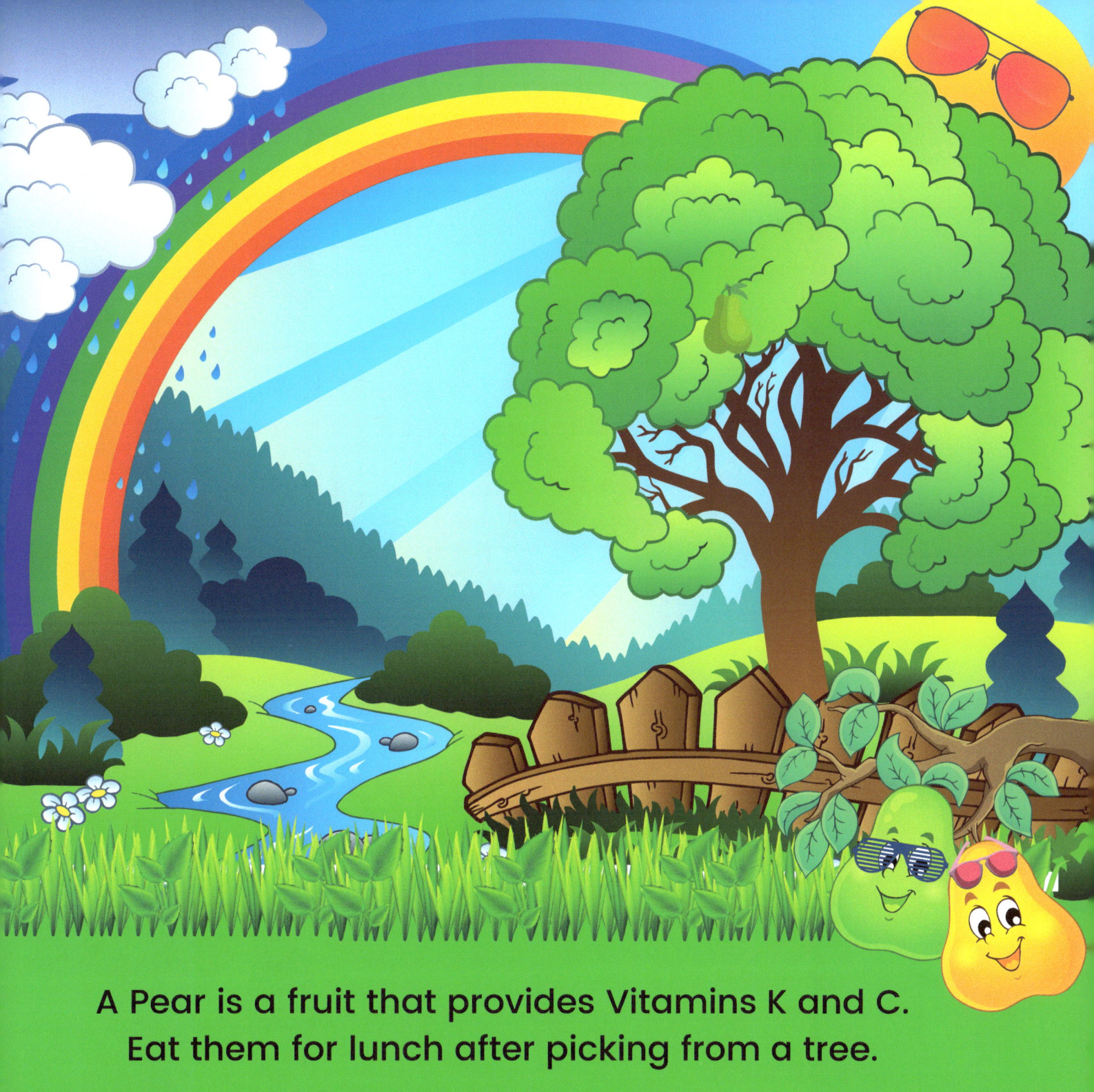

A Pear is a fruit that provides Vitamins K and C.
Eat them for lunch after picking from a tree.

Mr. Spinach lifts weights and is super-duper strong.
He goes by the nickname of Mr. HongKong.

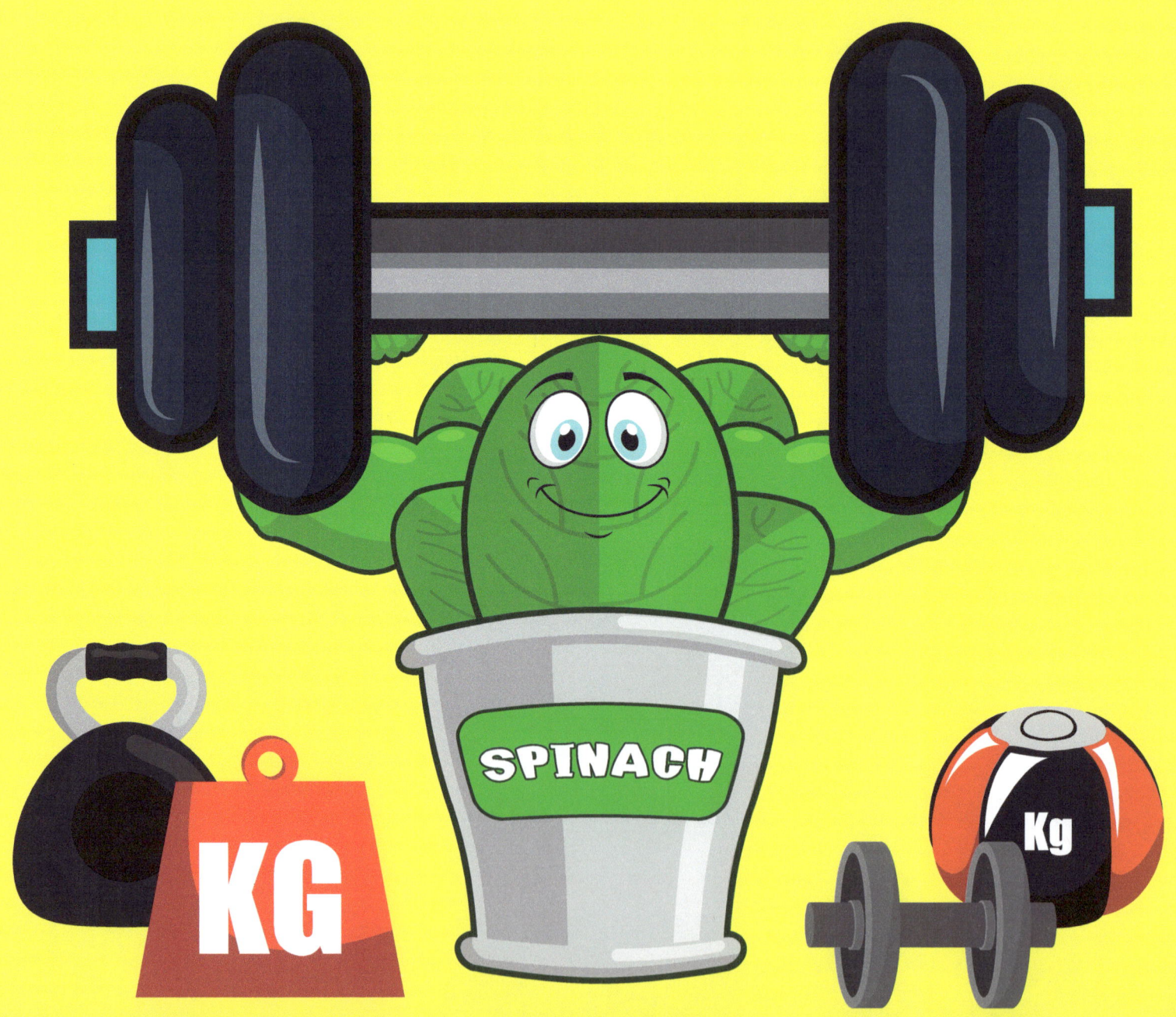

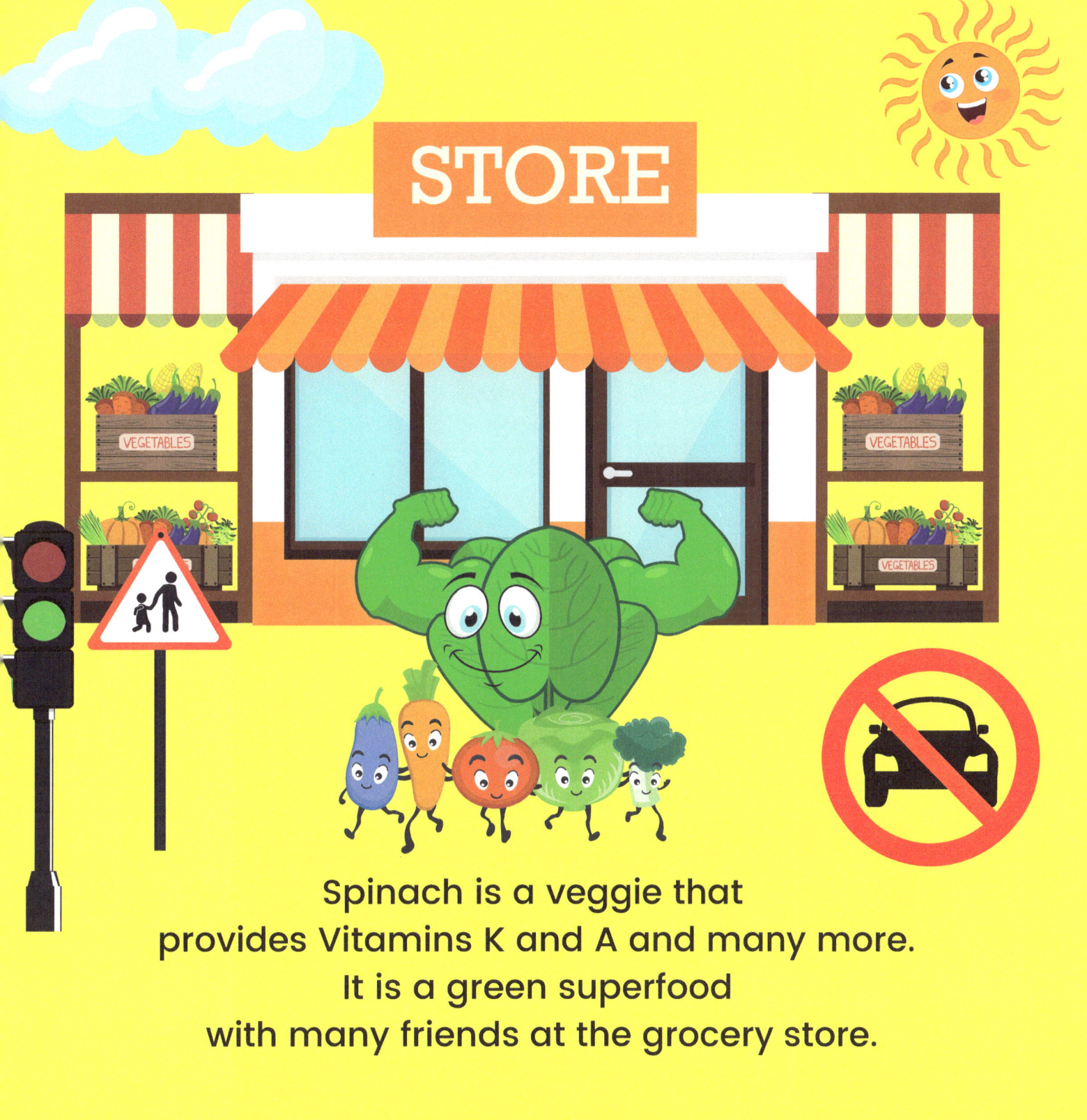

Spinach is a veggie that
provides Vitamins K and A and many more.
It is a green superfood
with many friends at the grocery store.

Green Celery was surprised on his 10th birthday
With lots of balloons and friends to play.

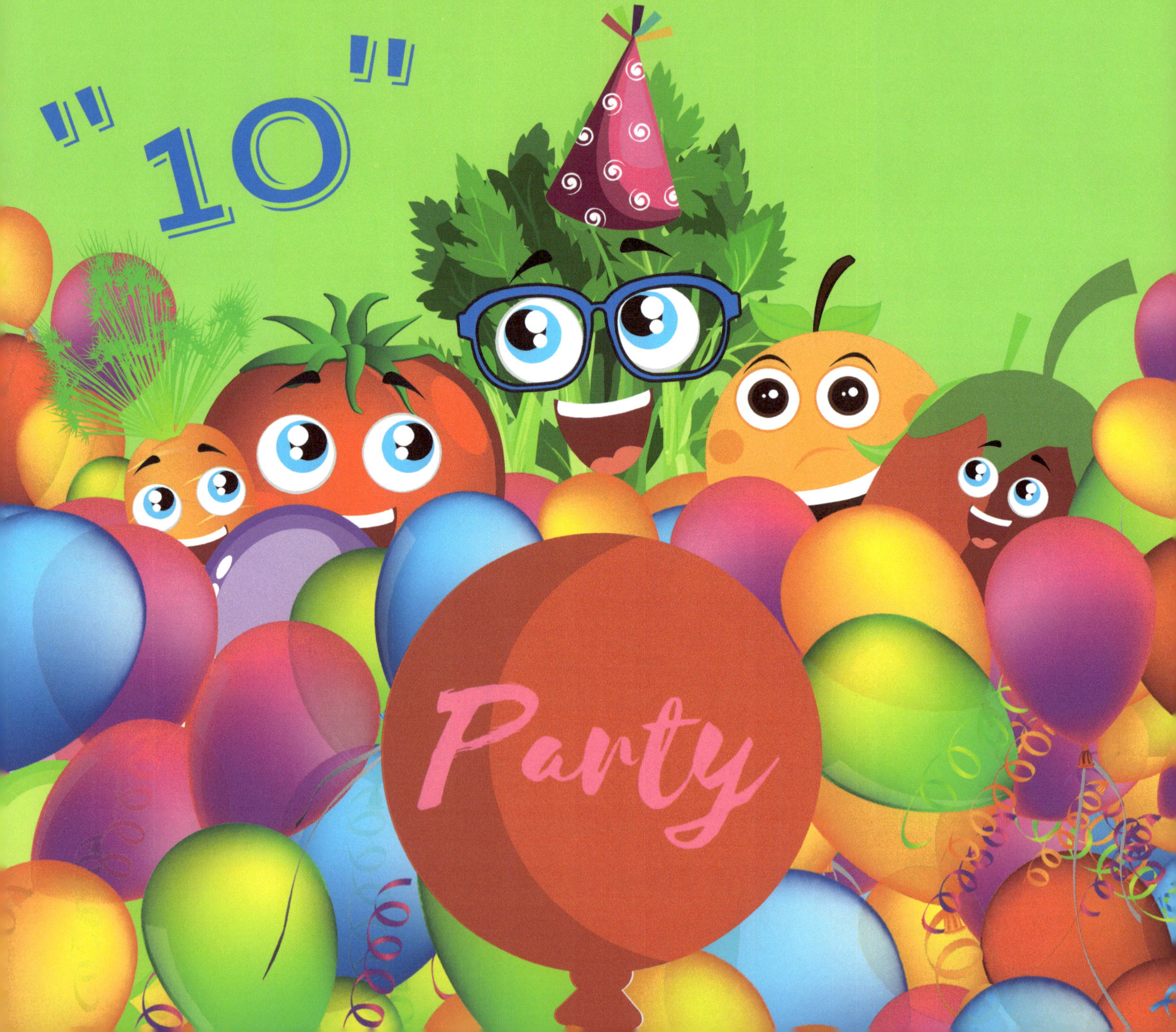

"10"

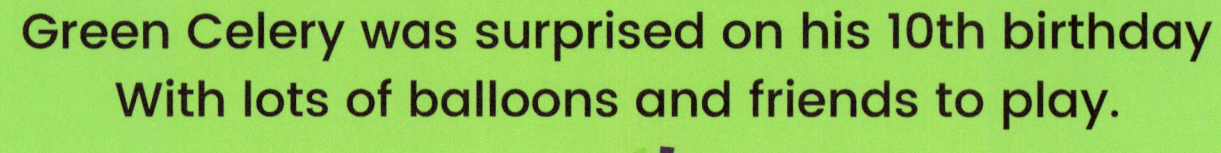

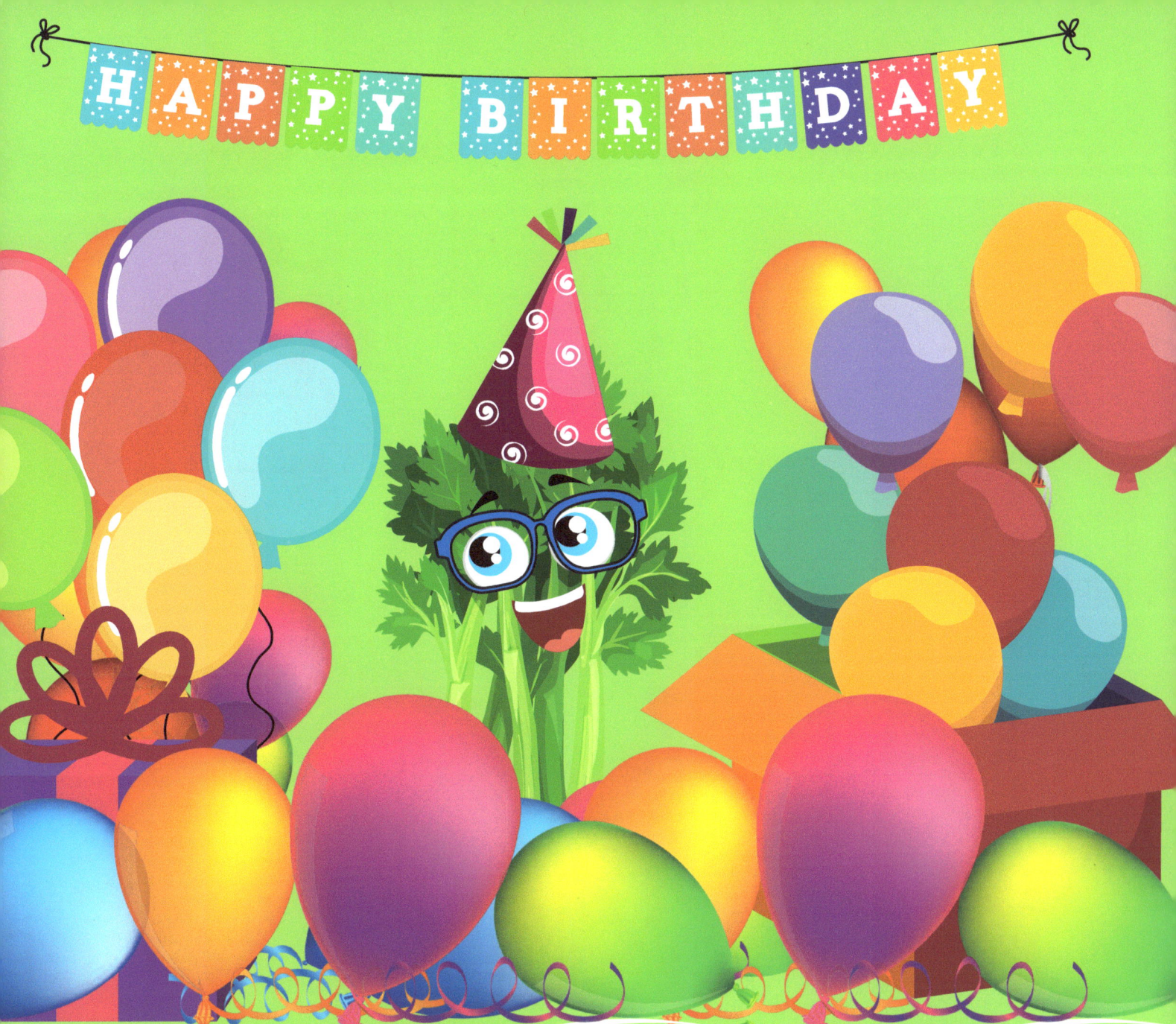

Celery is a veggie that provides Vitamins A, B, C and even K.
It is mostly water and helps to keep sickness away.

Orange Carrot and Red Apple will swim and have fun
Playing with the beach ball and bubble water gun.

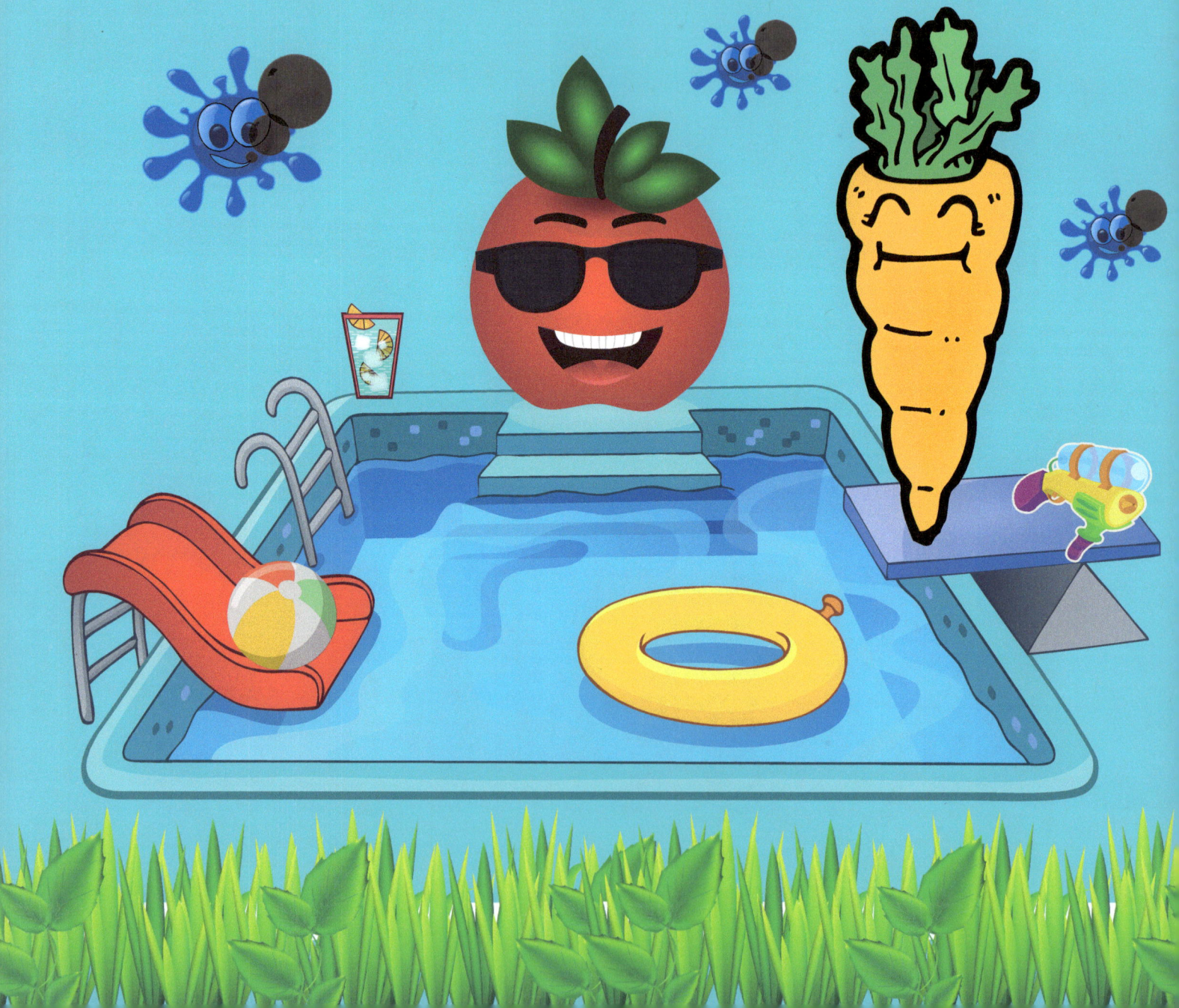

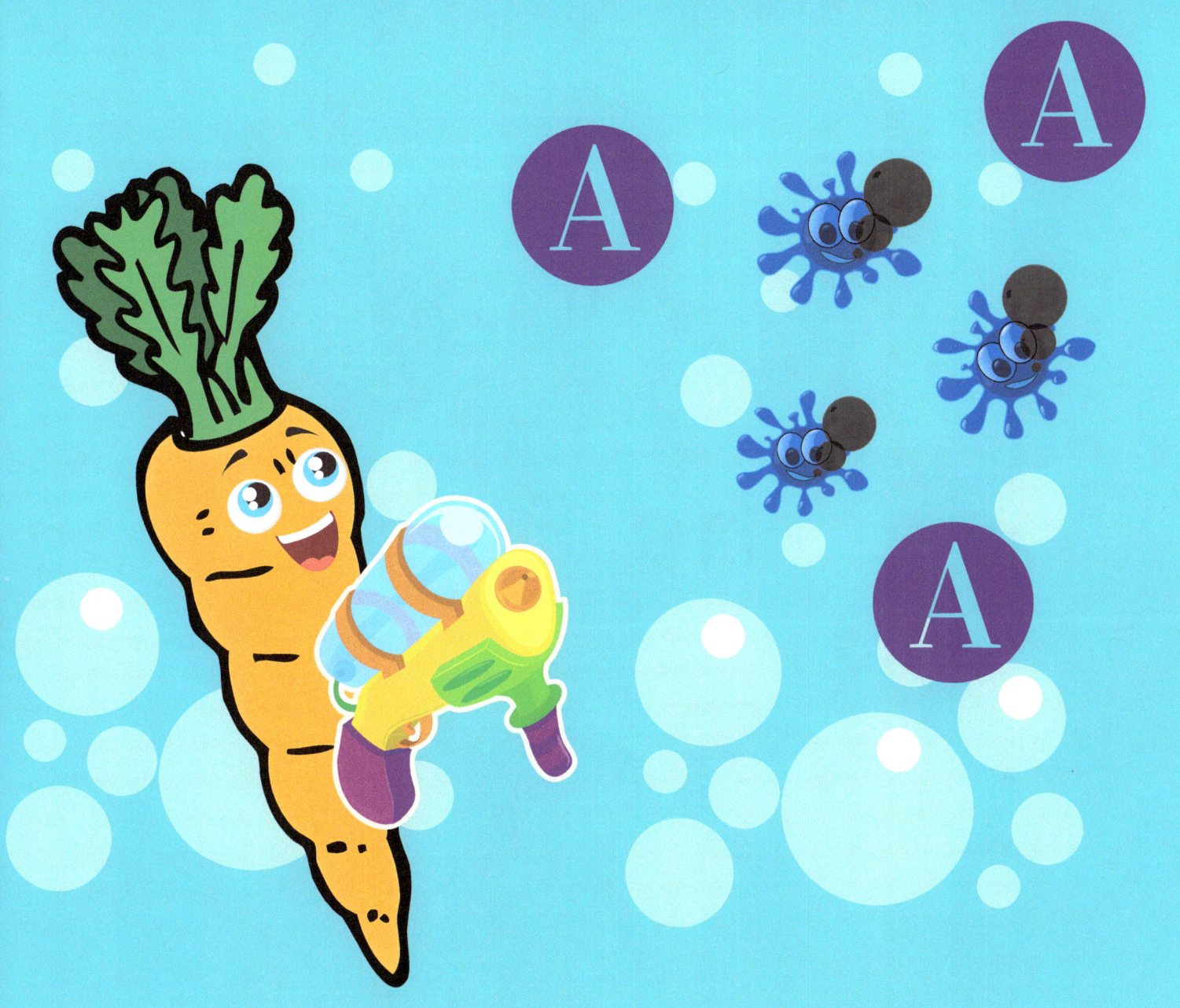

A Carrot is a veggie that provides Vitamin A.
It keeps the eyes healthy from day to day.

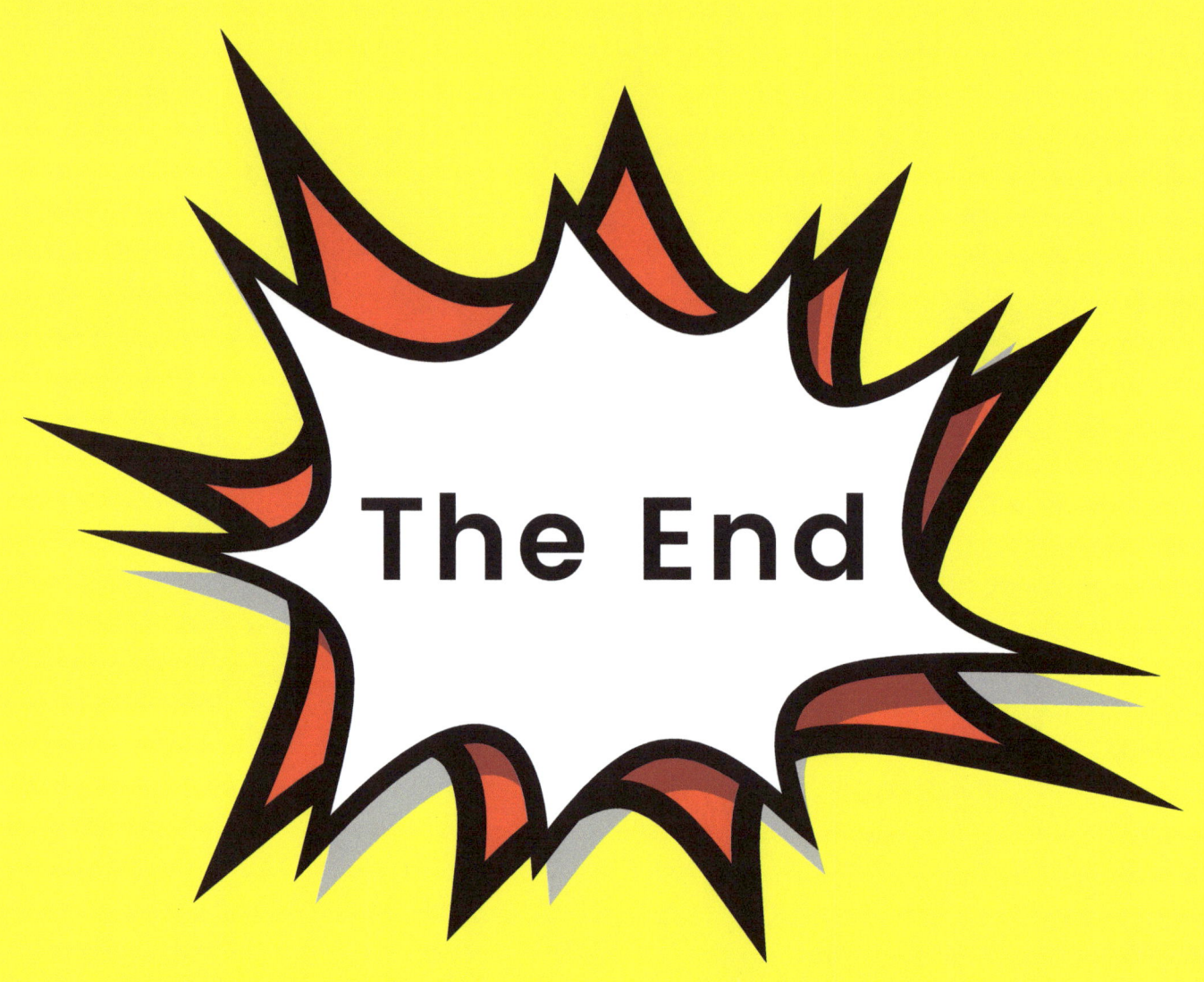

kidmotivation.com

About The Author

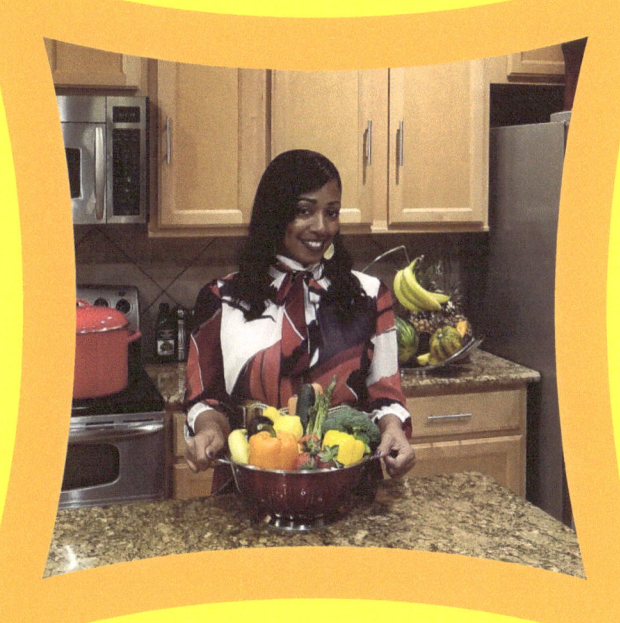

Tasana Scales is a Health & Wellness Advocate with 20 years experience as a Community Pharmacist. She advises a regimen rich in fruits and vegetables to reap healthy benefits and restore wellness. Tasana is married, has 3 kids and resides in the Dallas Suburbs.

Rhyming Story Words

- town / down
- car / star
- space / face

- sky / by
- play / way
- school / cool

- more / store
- vine / sunshine
- strong / HongKong

- fun / sun
- park / dark
- beach / peach

www.ingramcontent.com/pod-product-compliance
Lightning Source LLC
Chambersburg PA
CBHW041120070526
44584CB00002B/227